Awesome, Disgusting Science

GROSS SCIENCE OF FARTS AND BURPS

Stephanie Bearce

Black Rabbit Books

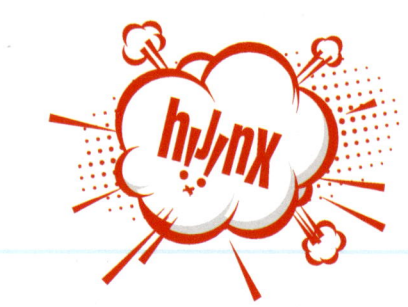

Hi Jinx is published by Black Rabbit Books
P.O. Box 227, Mankato, Minnesota, 56002.
www.blackrabbitbooks.com
Copyright © 2026 Black Rabbit Books

Alissa Thielges, editor; Jason Knudson, designer
and photo researcher

All rights reserved. No part of this book may
be reproduced in any form without written
permission from the publisher.

Library of Congress Cataloging-in-Publication Data
Names: Bearce, Stephanie author
Title: Gross science of farts and burps / by Stephanie Bearce.
Description: Mankato, MN : Black Rabbit Books, [2026] | Series: Awesome, disgusting science | Includes bibliographical references and index. | Audience: Ages 8-12 | Audience: Grades 4-6
Identifiers: LCCN 2025017485 (print) | LCCN 2025017486 (ebook) | ISBN 9781645824923 library binding | ISBN 9781645824985 paperback | ISBN 9781645825043 ebook
Subjects: LCSH: Flatulence—Juvenile literature | Belching—Juvenile literature
Classification: LCC RC862.F55 B43 2026 (print) | LCC RC862.F55 (ebook) | DDC 612.3/2—dc23/eng/20250811
LC record available at https://lccn.loc.gov/2025017485
LC ebook record available at https://lccn.loc.gov/2025017486"

Printed in the United States of America.

Image Credits
Freepik/AI Image Creator, cover, 1, brgfx, 3, 14, 23, freepik, 17, 21, grelectric, cover, 1, 5, 6, 8, 9, 12, 13, 20, macrovector, cover, 1, 5, pch.vector, 8, ssstocker, 2, 3, 14, 15, 23, upklyak, 12, 13; Shutterstock/Andrea Izzotti, 12-13, Anton Brand, 18, Bohbeh creations, 10, Catherine Lall, 19, Damsea, 12, Dennis Forster, 11, JocularityArt, 9, Kichigin, 11, Krakenimages.com, 4, Marko Aliaksandr, 7, Memo Angeles, 20, MemoryMan, 15, Mike_shots, 18-19, mybox, 7, tonsky, 15, Yankovsky88, 8, 32 pixels, 4-5; Wikimedia Commons/Katja Schulz, 16, Melissa McMasters, 16.

<small>Every effort has been made to contact copyright holders for material reproduced in this book. Any omissions will be rectified in subsequent printings if notice is given to the publisher.</small>

CONTENTS

CHAPTER 1
Stinky Science.........5

CHAPTER 2
The Experiments......6

CHAPTER 3
Get in on the Hi Jinx..20

Other Resources...........22

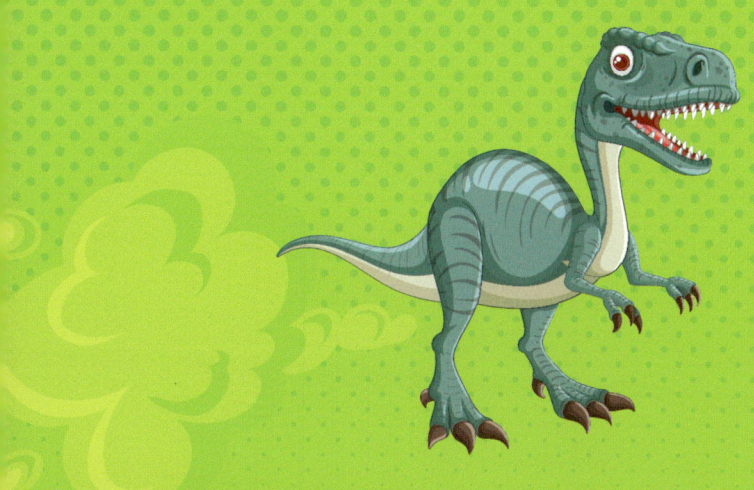

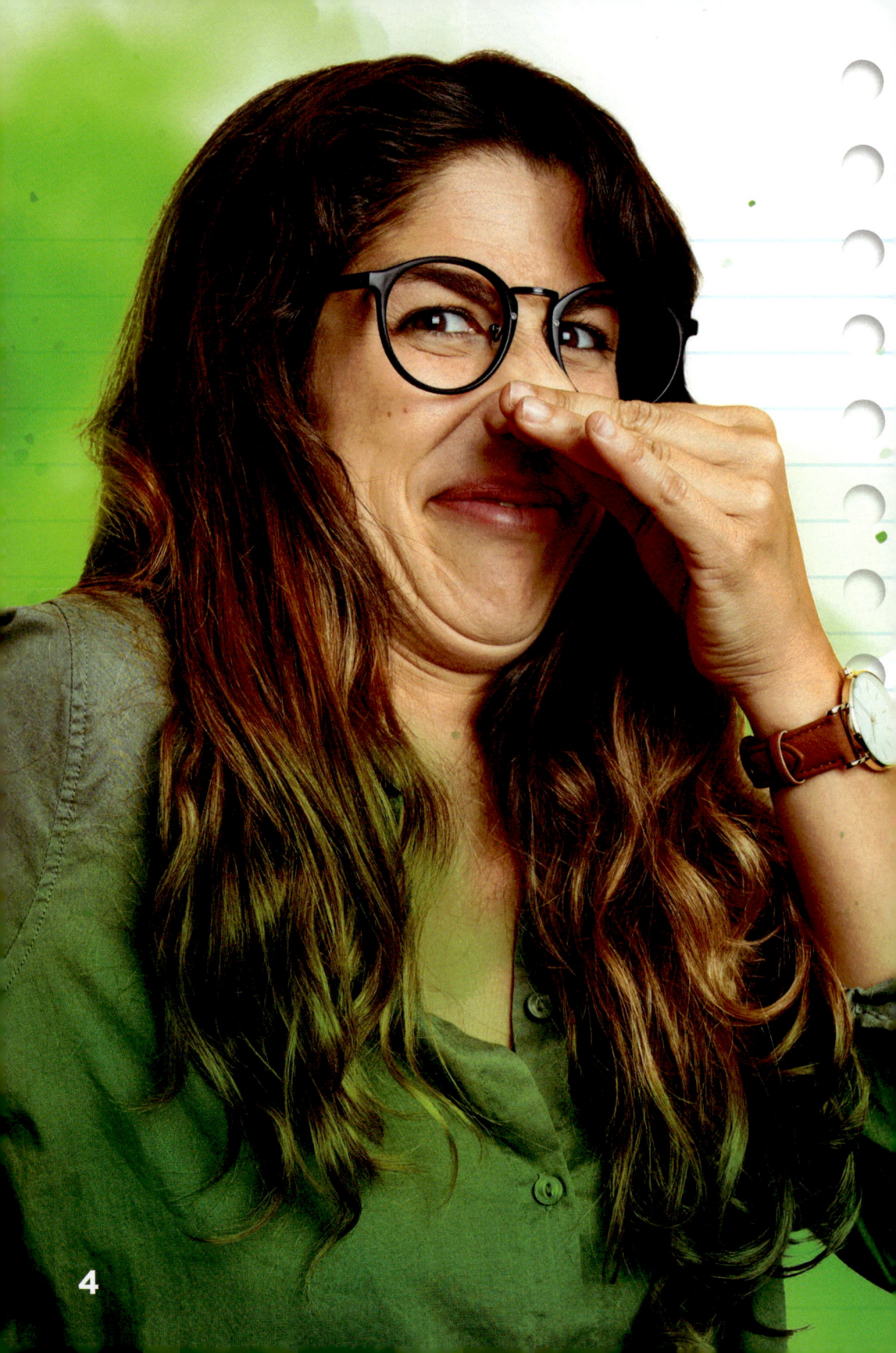

Chapter 1
STINKY SCIENCE

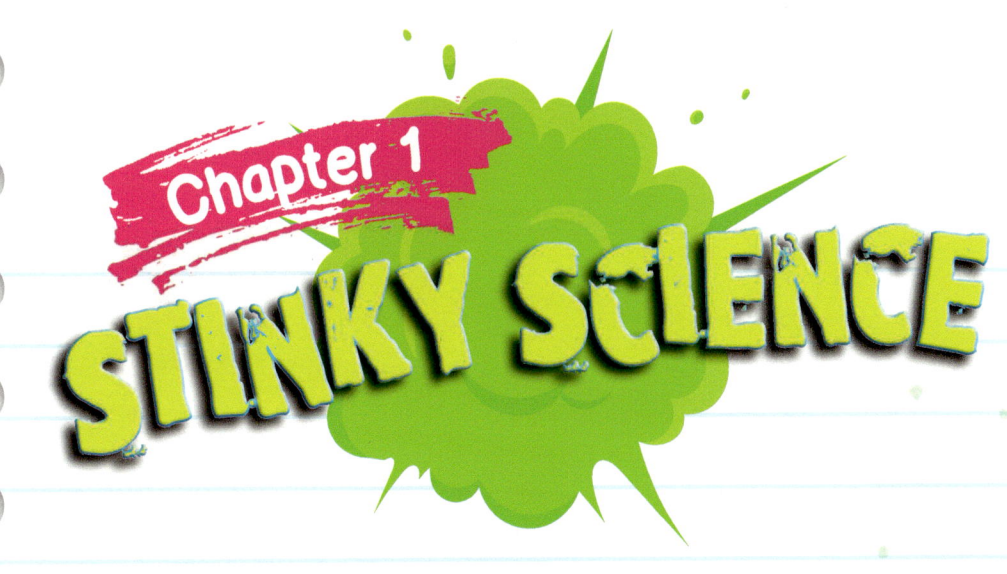

PHHHttt! Whoa, what's that stink? Did you fart? Probably. Every creature with a **digestive system** farts. **Bacteria** give off gas as they break down food. The gas comes out as farts and burps. And the stink? That's the smell of your gut. Dive into this stench in the name of science!

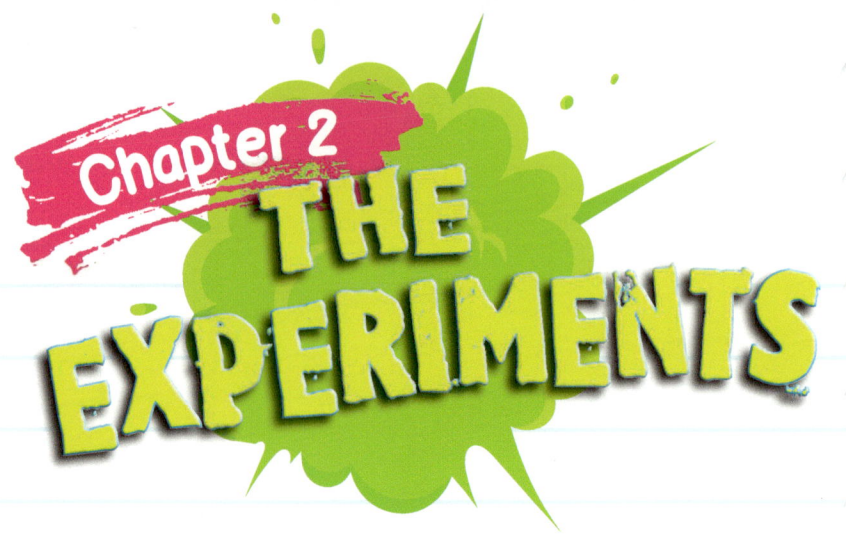

Chapter 2: THE EXPERIMENTS

Fart Collectors

Have you ever tried to capture a fart? Scientists did this! They made a sensor that someone can swallow. It slides through the **intestines**. It sniffs out signs of gas. It sends the **data** to a computer. Then the small sensor is pooped out. Scientists learn what a "healthy" fart contains. This is important to gut health.

Scientists say it is not good to hold in a fart. Let it rip!

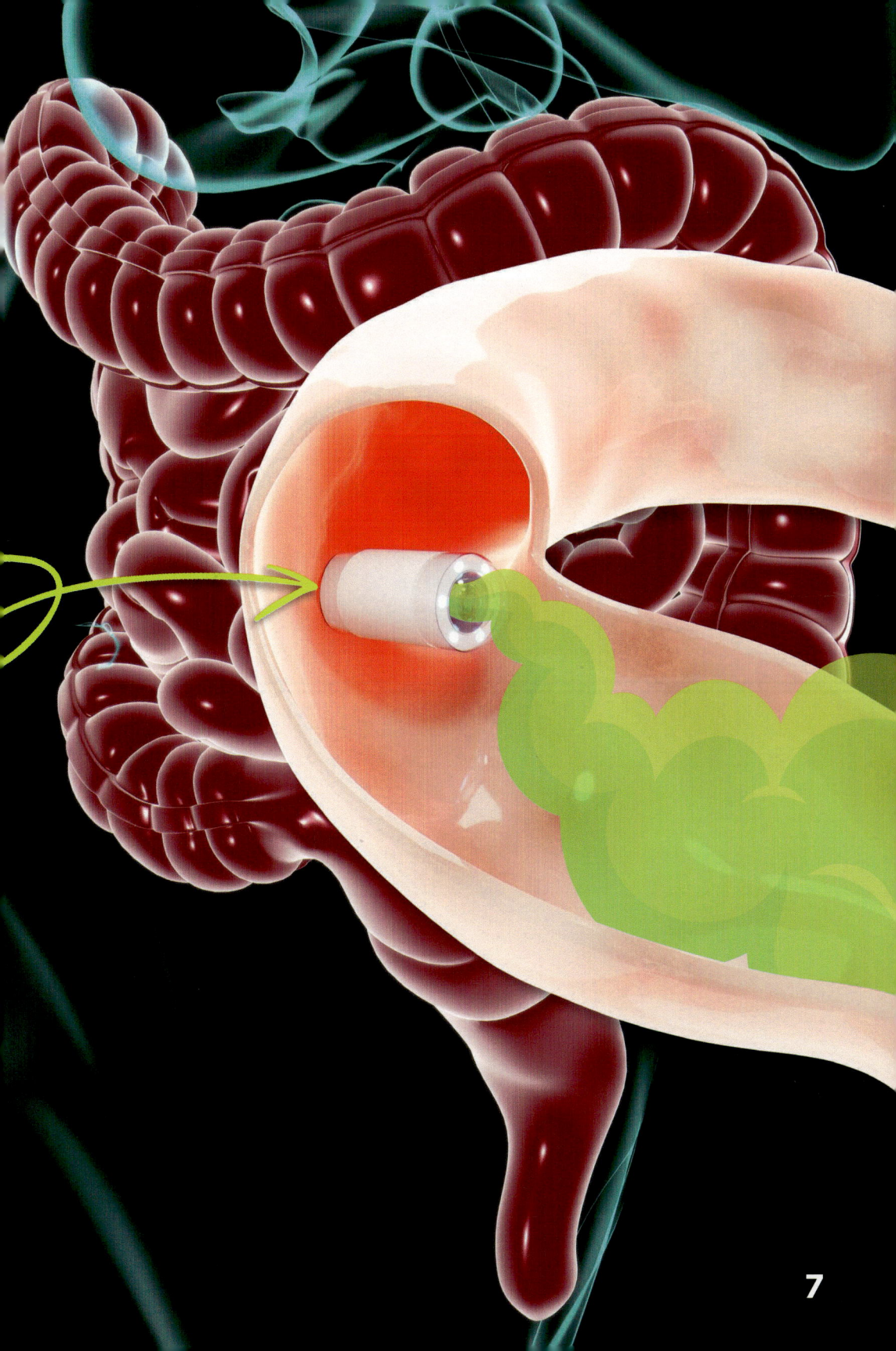

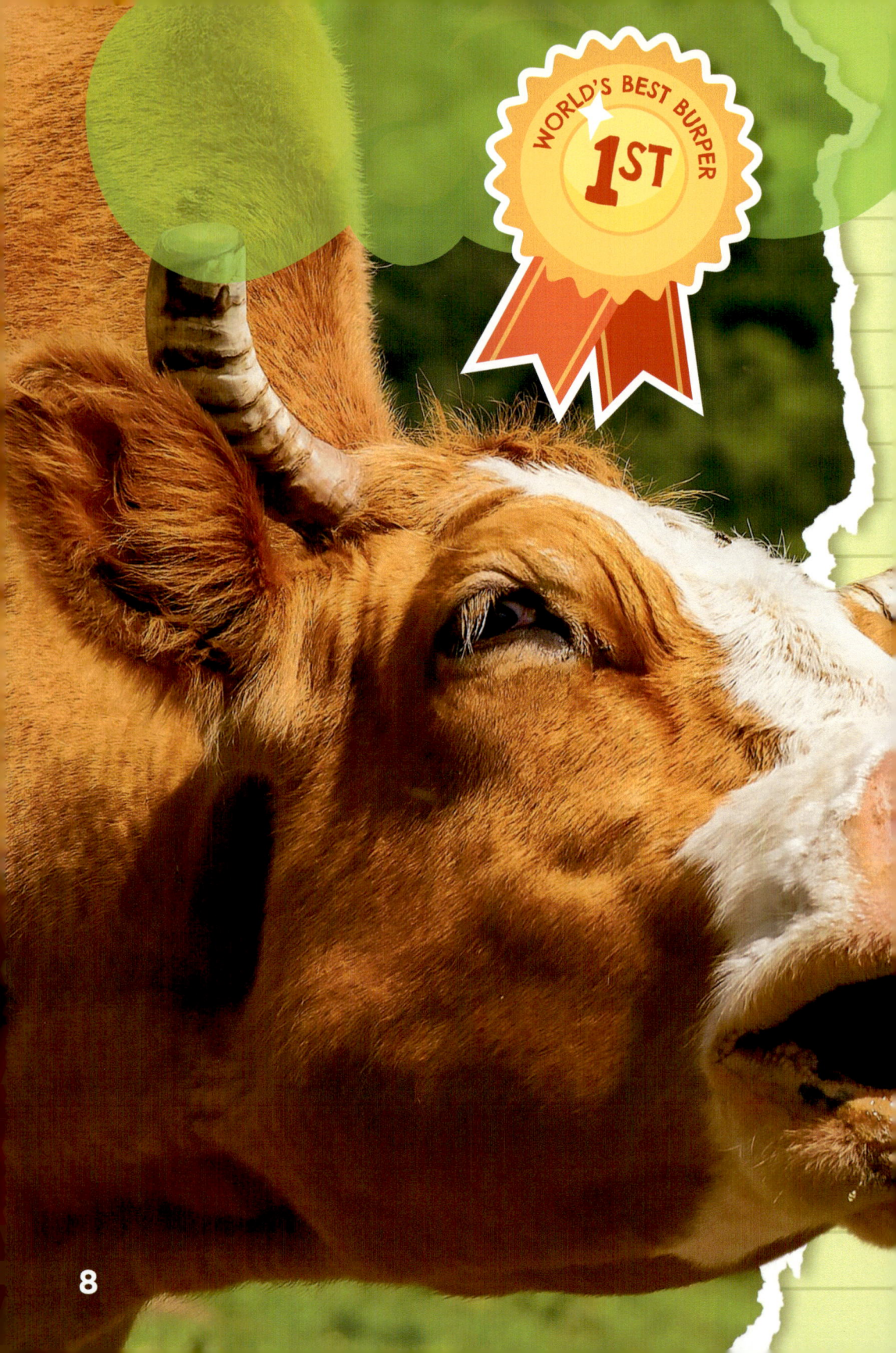

Queen of Burps

Imagine a world championship for burping. Who would win? Cows! They burp about every 90 seconds. That's 960 burps a day! Scientists want to stop this gassiness. Cows burp methane. This gas warms the planet. Scientists study what cows eat. Different food might help. Fighting **climate change**, one burp at a time!

A big word for farts is flatulence.

Fart Talk

How would you like to talk by farting? That would be one stinky chat! Herring fish might communicate this way. Scientists put microphones under water. They listened and watched. They heard popping sounds. Then bubbles came from the fish's butts. This seemed to help the herring swim together. They could be talking with farts!

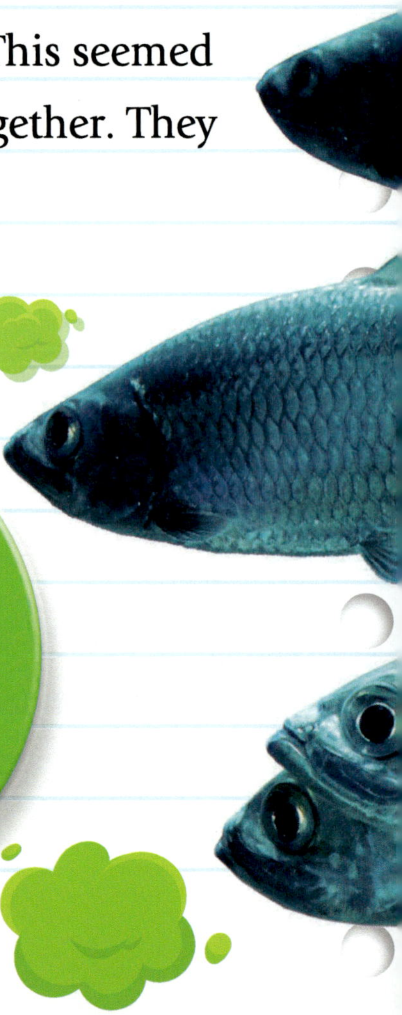

Scientists called the sounds "fast repetitive ticks" (FRTs). They happened mostly at night.

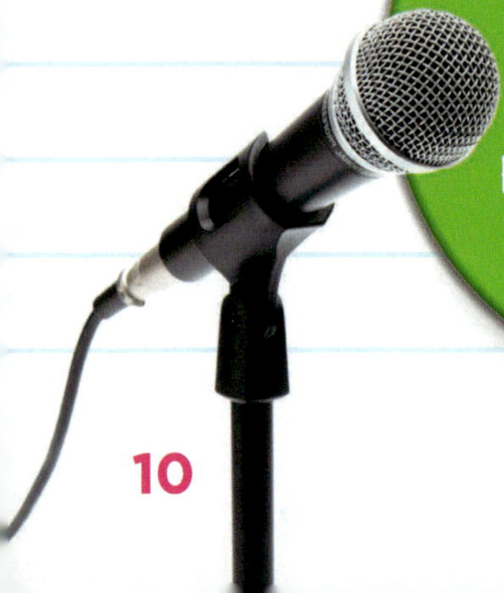

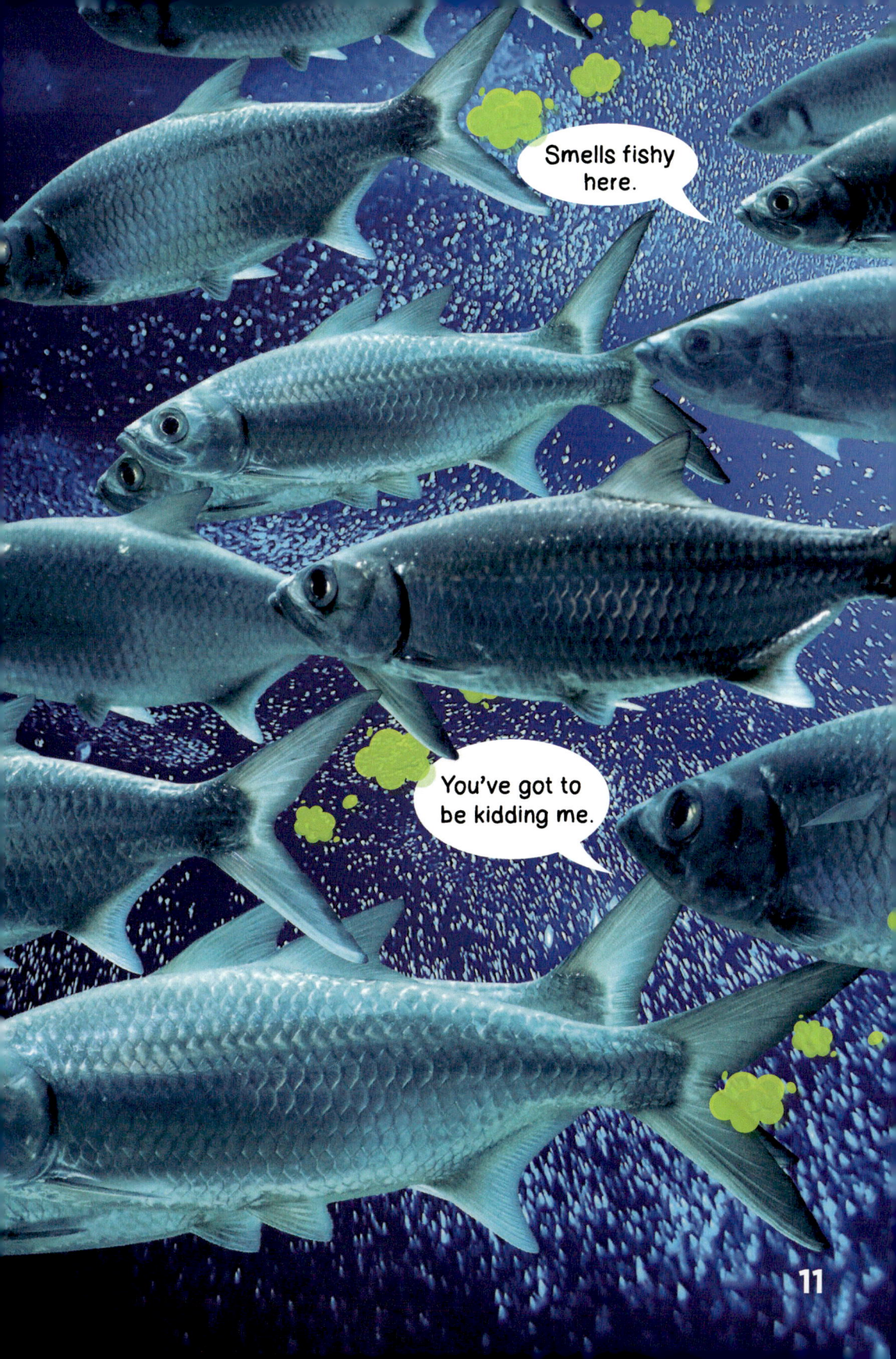

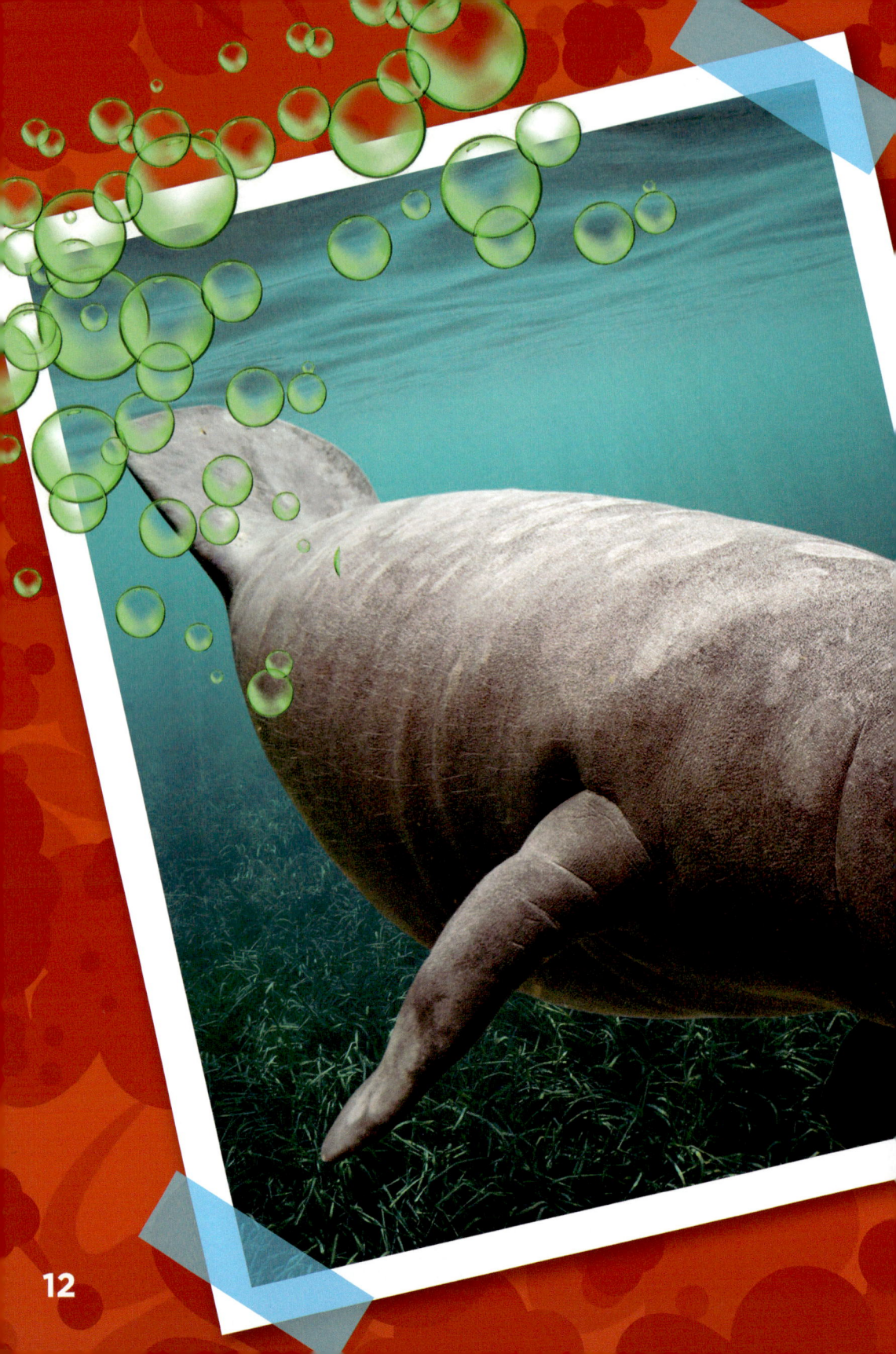

Fart or Float?

Did you know manatees use farts to swim? They store extra gas in their intestines. This helps them float. And when they want to dive? They fart! They get rid of the extra gas and are heavy.

Scientists studied manatee **anatomy**. They learned these animals have a strong diaphragm. It helps them control their farting.

Mound Defense

Termites are tiny. But they pack a powerful fart. They spew out 20 million tons (18 million metric tons) of methane every year! That's a lot of gas. Scientists worried this would harm our planet. They tested different termite mounds. They found much of the gas disappeared. The mound cleaned it up. Awesome!

Dinosaurs were the biggest farters ever. They farted so much they might have created a warmer world!

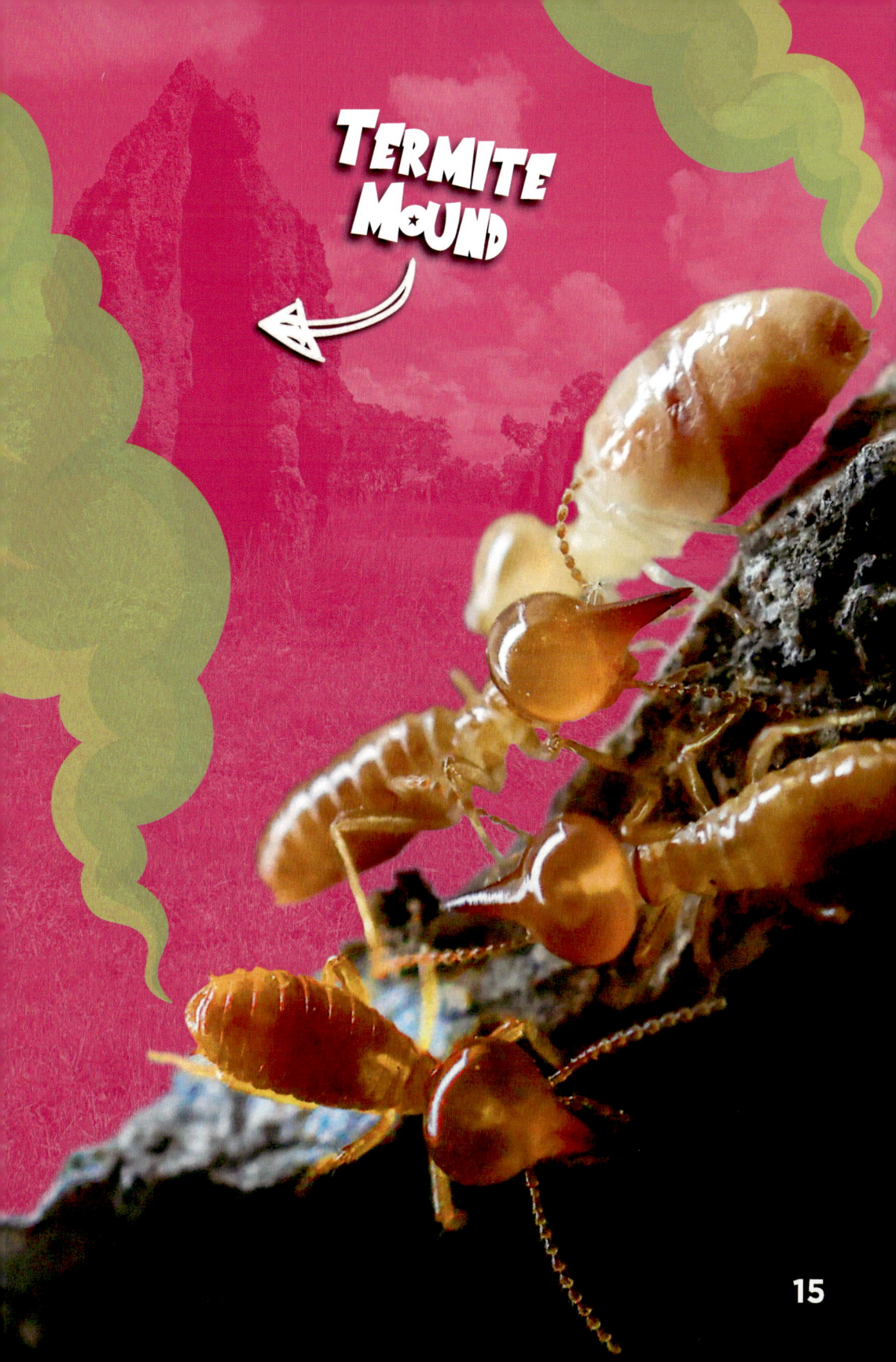

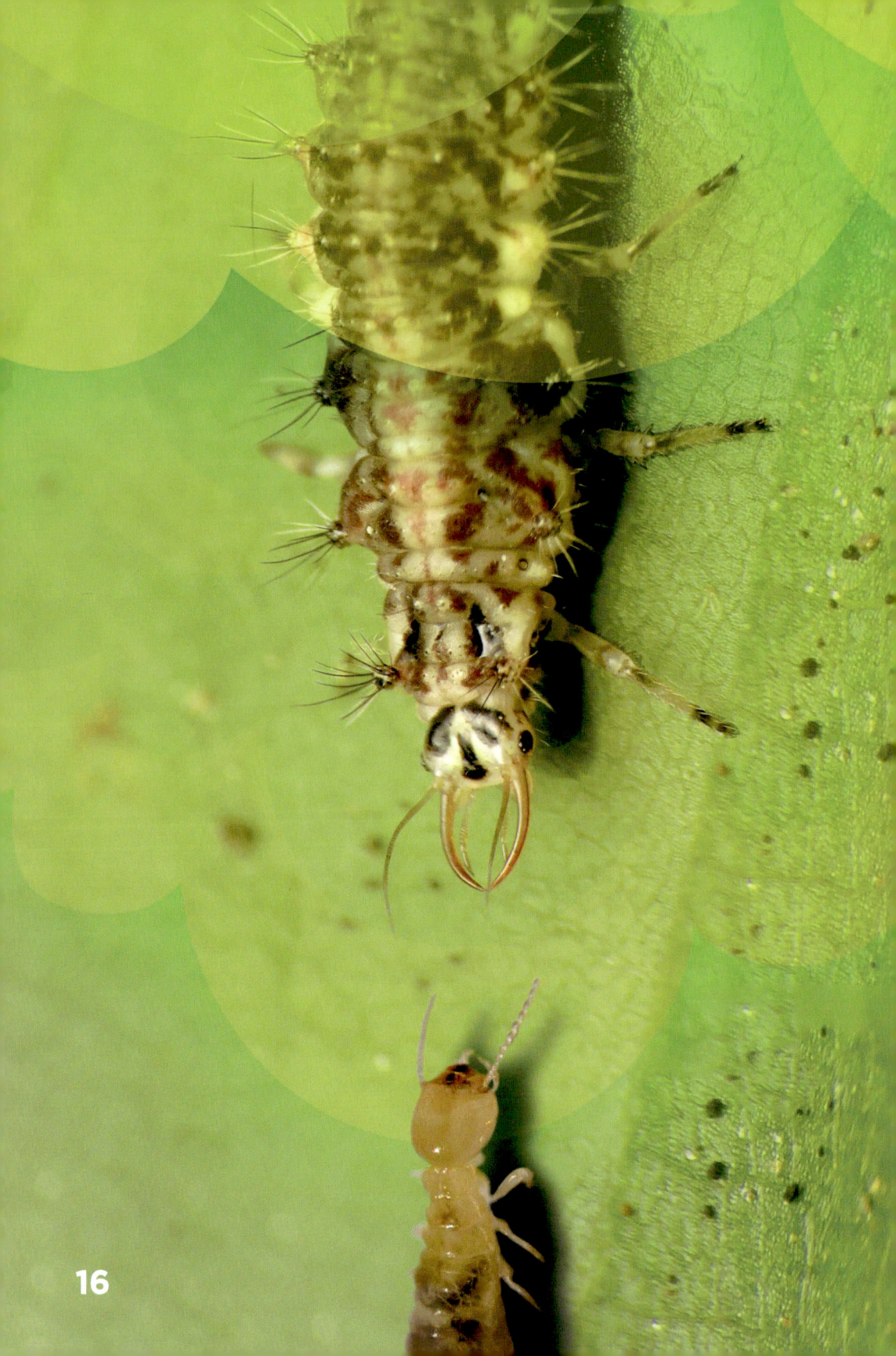

Killer Farts

Can farts be deadly? Yes! Lacewing insect **larva** hatch near termite mounds. The tiny larva come out hungry. And they have a secret weapon. They use poison farts to kill termites. Then they feast on the bodies. Scientists are experimenting with this idea. They want to make a natural termite killer.

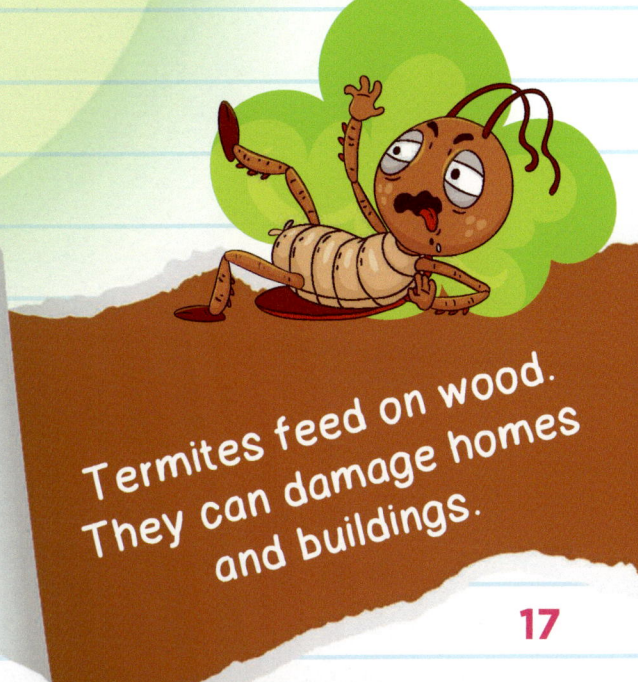

Termites feed on wood. They can damage homes and buildings.

Space Burps

Burping in space is a terrible idea. Astronauts have proved it. On Earth, **gravity** helps you burp. The gas rises to the top of your stomach. Gas comes up, food stays down. But in zero gravity? The liquids and gasses mix like a chunky stew. Try to burp, and boom—surprise puke! Hope you like helmet soup.

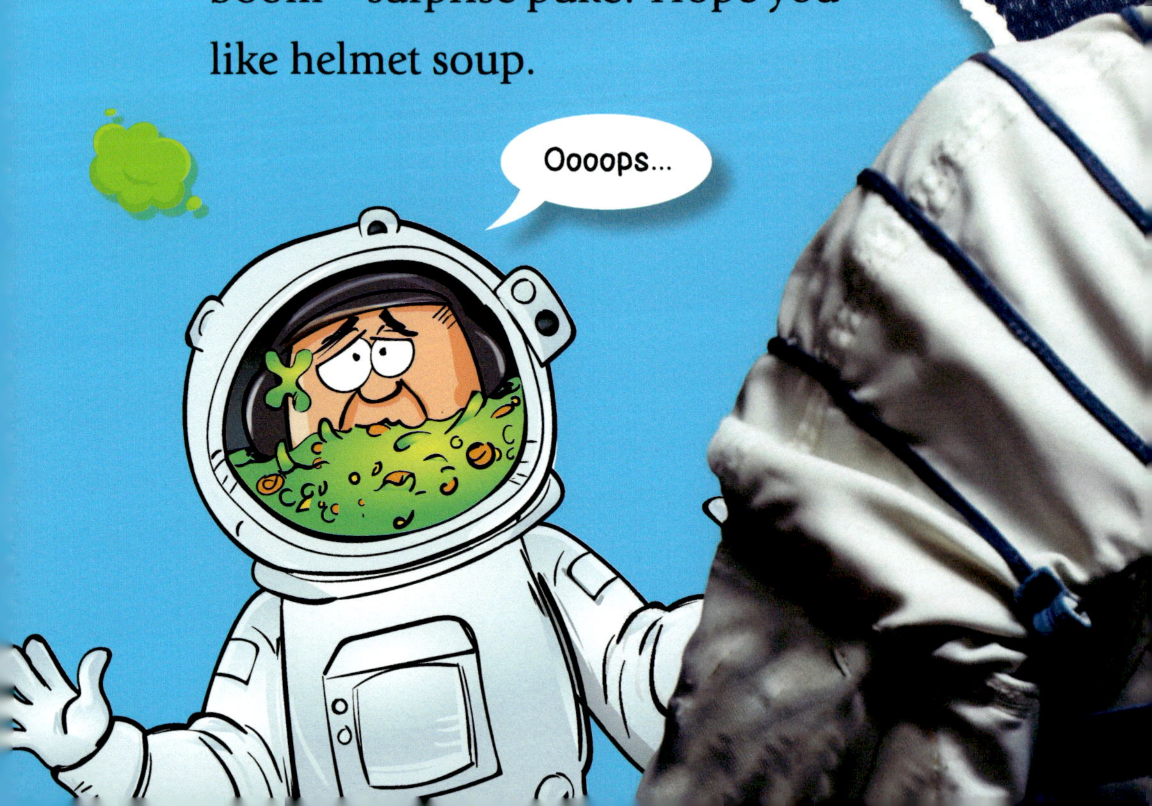

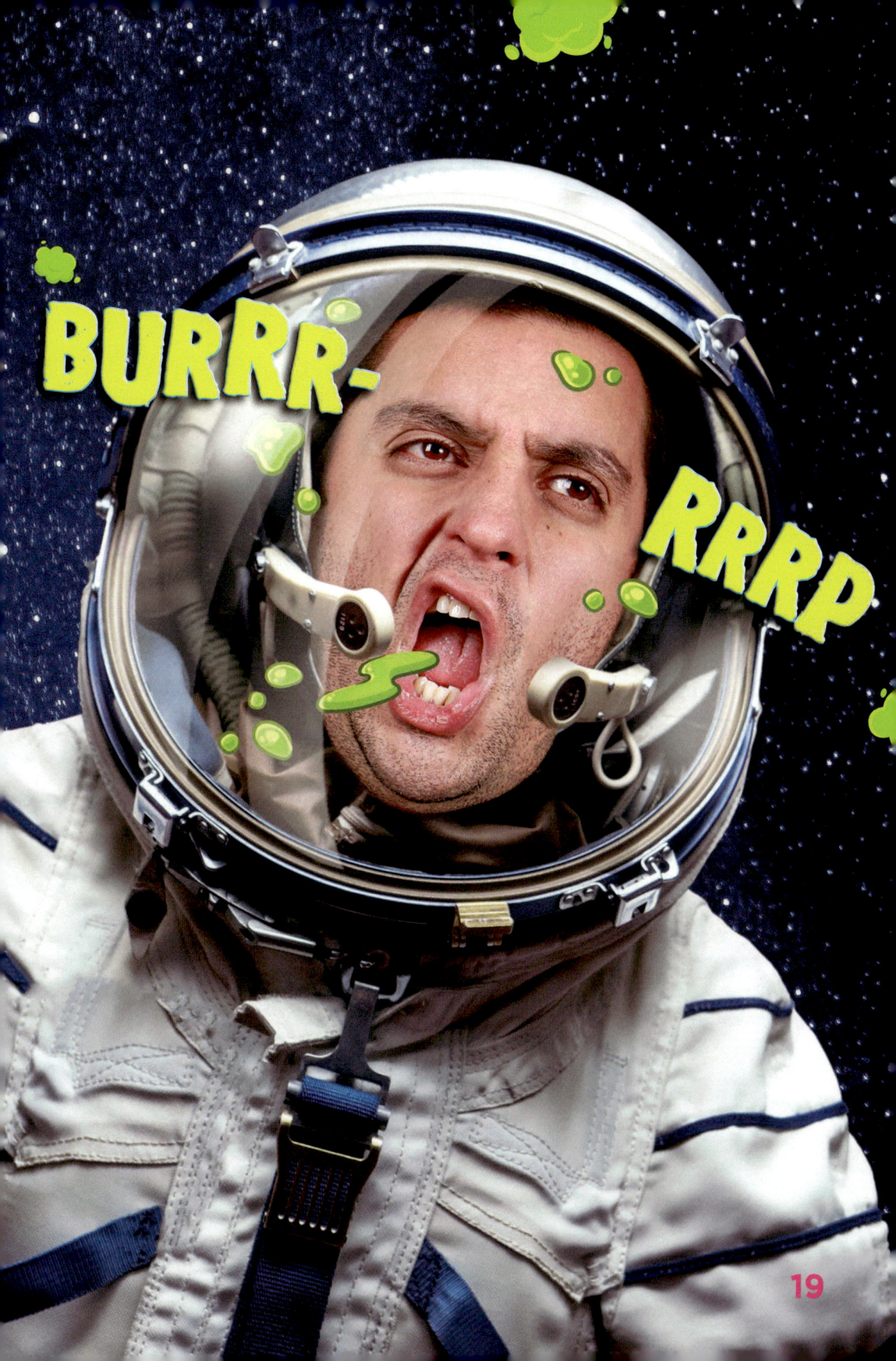

Chapter 3
GET IN ON THE HI JINX

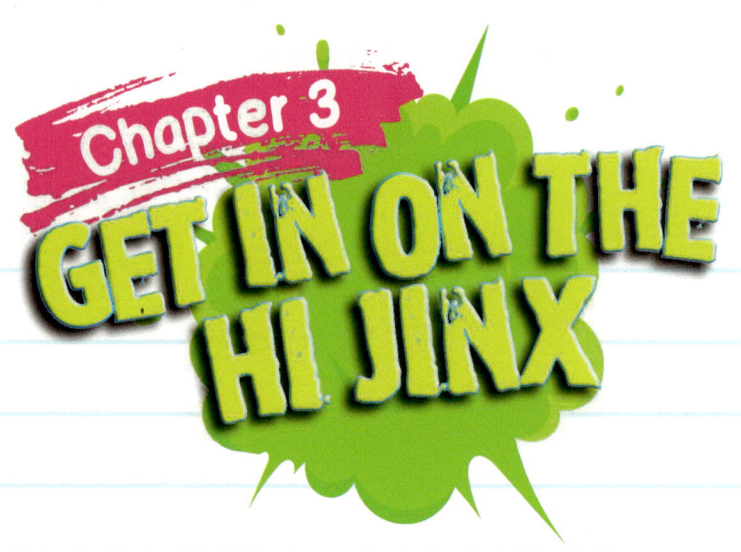

Love nature and wildlife? Become a **conservation** assistant! They collect data and watch animal behavior—including farts and burps! No college degree is needed. Training programs can help you get started. You'll get hands-on experience. You can discover new awesomely disgusting facts!

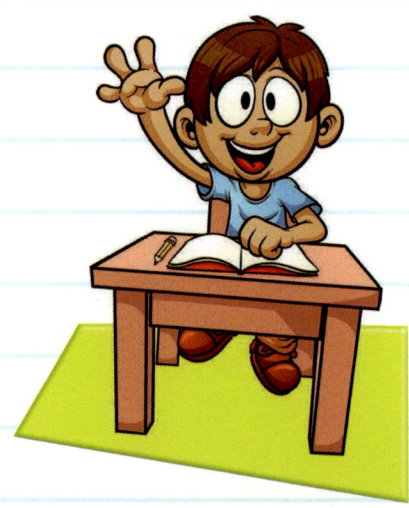

Take It One Step More

1. What makes farts stinky? Research to find out!

2. What other ways do animals use their farts in the wild?

3. If you were a scientist, would you want to study farts and burps? Can think of your own experiment?

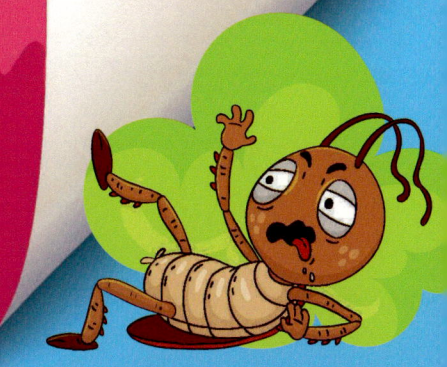

GLOSSARY

anatomy (uh-NAT-uh-mee)—the parts that form a living thing

bacteria (bak-TEER-ee-uh)—a small living thing

climate change (KLAHY-mit CHEYNJ)—changes in the Earth's weather patterns

conservation (kon-ser-vey-shuhn)—the protection of animals, plants, and natural resources

data (DAT-uh)—information created or stored by a computer

digestive system (dy-JES-tive)—the organs in a body that break down food into energy and get rid of waste

gravity (GRAV-i-tee)—the natural force that pulls physical things toward each other

intestines (en-TE-stenz)—the part of the digestive system where most food is digested

larva (LAR-vuh)—the wormlike form of an animal that hatches from an egg

LEARN MORE

BOOKS

Branzei, Sylvia. *Grossology: The Science of Really Gross Things!* New York: Grosset & Dunlap, 2025.

Humphrey, Natalie. *Cow's Fart!* Buffalo, New York: Gareth Stevens Publishing, 2024.

Stiefel, Chana. *How Rude!: Animals that Burp, Toot, Spit, and Screetch to Survive.* New York: Union Square Kids, 2026.

WEBSITES

Could You Fart Your Way to the Moon?
tpt.pbslearningmedia.org/resource/could-you-fart-your-pbs-space-time/could-you-fart-your-way-to-the-moon-video-pbs-space-time/

Why Do I Burp?
www.wonderopolis.org/wonder/Why-Do-I-Burp

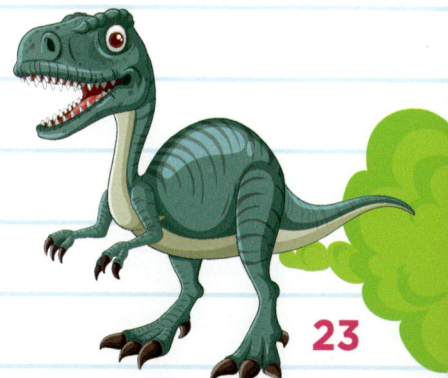

INDEX

A

astronauts, 18

C

communication, 10

conservation assistants, 20

cows, 9

D

dinosaurs, 14

G

global warming, 9, 14

I

insect larvae, 17

M

manatees, 13

methane gas, 9, 14

S

sensors, 6

T

termites, 14, 17